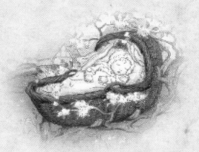

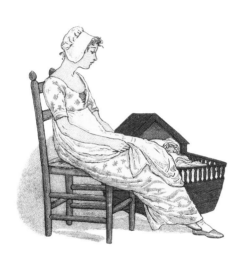

THE
KATE GREENAWAY

FIRST YEAR
BABY BOOK

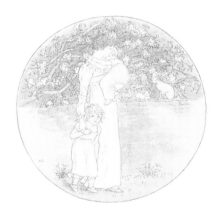

SHELDRAKE PRESS
LONDON

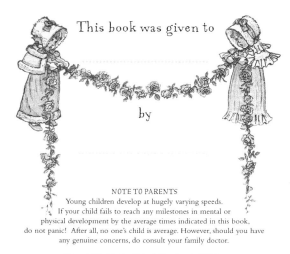

This book was given to

by

NOTE TO PARENTS

Young children develop at hugely varying speeds.
If your child fails to reach any milestones in mental or
physical development by the average times indicated in this book,
do not panic! After all, no one's child is average. However, should you have
any genuine concerns, do consult your family doctor.

First published in the United Kingdom in 1999 by
Sheldrake Press, 188 Cavendish Road, London, SW12 0DA

Devised in association with Rosemary Rigge, physiotherapist and mother of three, Grad. Dip. Phys.,
M.C.S.P., S.R.P., and Mary Farman, midwife and nurse, R.S.C.N., R.N., R.M.

Edited by Simon Rigge and Cristina Lipscomb
Designed by Ivor Claydon Graphics

Origination, printing and binding in Singapore under the supervision of
MRM Graphics Ltd, Winslow, Bucks.

ISBN 1 873329 30 X

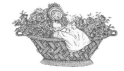

FIRST SIGNS OF LIFE

Confirmation of pregnancy ....

First person told ....

First scan ....

Scan photograph

First heart-beat heard ....

First kick felt ....

First names considered ....

....

....

....

FIRST DAY

Birth . . . .

Time . . . .

Date . . . .

Place . . . .

Weight . . . .

Length . . . .

Eye colour . . . .

Hair colour . . . .

Birthmarks . . . .

Resemblances . . . .

Doctor . . . .

Midwife . . . .

General practitioner . . . .

First feed . . . .

First visitors . . . .

. . . .

First gifts and cards . . . .

. . . .

. . . .

FIRST PHOTOGRAPH

Photograph

FIRST HEALTH CHECKS

AT BIRTH:

Apgar score ....

    colour ....

    heart rate ....

    muscle tone ....

    breathing ....

    crying ....

WITHIN 24 HOURS:

First health check by paediatrician or GP

....

....

6TH OR 7TH DAY AFTER BIRTH:

Guthrie test ....

....

AT 6 WEEKS:

Hearing test ....

....

....

FIRST VACCINATIONS

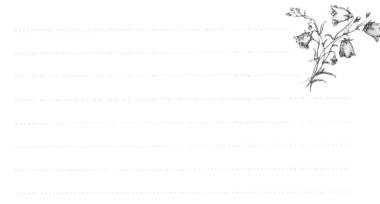

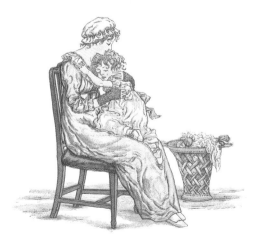

FIRST DAY HOME

First car ride

First address

First feed

First clothes

First cot

First maternity nurse

First visitors

First toys

First night

FIRST RITES

Christening or naming ....

....

Full name ....

Date ....

Place ....

Godparents ....

....

Guests ....

....

....

....

Gifts ....

....

....

....

....

FIRST TOILETTE

First bath at home ....

First nail-cut ....

First hair-cut ....

Lock of hair

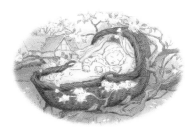

FIRST THREE MONTHS

Weight ....

Date ....

Feeding ....

Sleep pattern ....

....

....

Health visitor ....

General progress

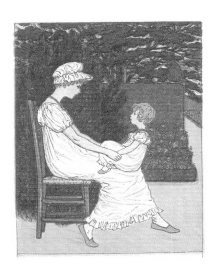

....

....

....

Character

....

....

....

13

FIRST HAND PRINT

FIRST FOOT PRINT

FIRST MEALS

AT 4 MONTHS:

First solids

FROM 6 TO 9 MONTHS:

First meal in a highchair

BY 12 MONTHS:

First drink from a cup or tumbler

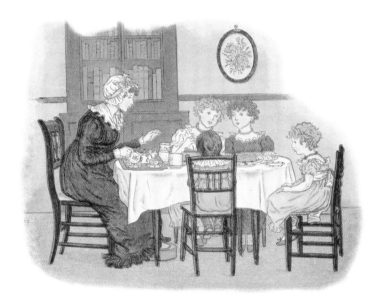

FIRST EXPRESSIONS

FROM BIRTH TO 6 MONTHS:

First smile ....

....

First laugh ....

....

First tears ....

....

FROM 6 TO 9 MONTHS:

First clear syllable ....

....

First expression in front of a mirror ....

....

First response to own name ....

....

First signs of imitation ....

....

....

From 9 to 12 months:

First wave bye-bye ....

....

First clap of hands ....

....

First understanding of 'no' and 'bye-bye' ....

....

....

First babbling of 'mama', 'dada' ....

....

....

First meaningful word ....

....

....

FIRST SIX MONTHS

Weight ....

Date ....

Sleep pattern ....

....

....

General progress ....

....

....

....

....

....

....

....

....

....

....

Character

FIRST TEETH

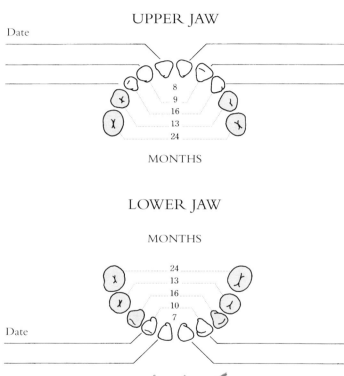

UPPER JAW

Date

8
9
16
13
24

MONTHS

LOWER JAW

MONTHS

24
13
16
10
7

Date

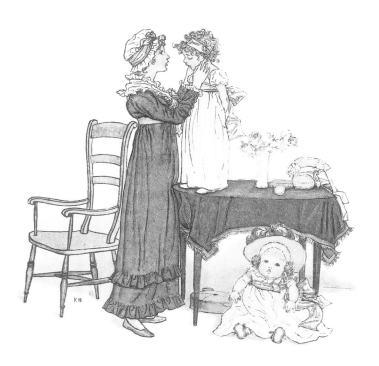

FIRST STEPS IN PHYSICAL DEVELOPMENT

FROM 3 TO 6 MONTHS:

First time holds head up ....

First time holds object ....

First time rolls over ....

FROM 6 TO 12 MONTHS:

First time puts foot to mouth ....

First full night's sleep ....

First crawl ....

FROM 9 TO 18 MONTHS:

First unsupported sit ....

First aided walk ....

....

First unaided walk ....

....

First grasp with index finger and thumb ....

....

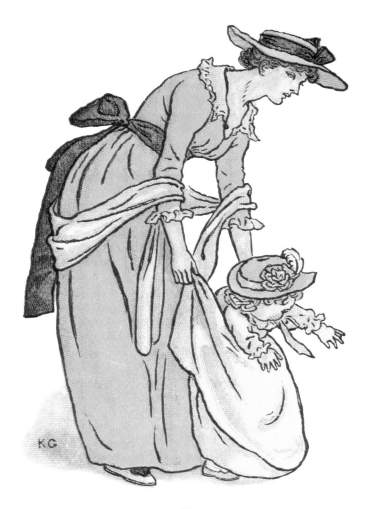

FIRST NINE MONTHS

Weight . . . .

Date . . . .

Sleep pattern . . . .

. . . .

. . . .

General progress . . . .

. . . .

. . . .

. . . .

. . . .

. . . .

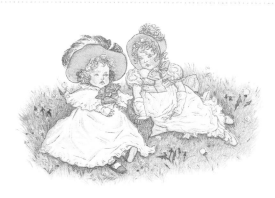

Character

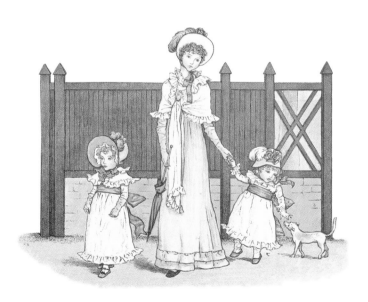

FIRST ENTERTAINMENTS

First lullaby

First playmate

First outing in pram/push-chair

First playgroup

First holiday

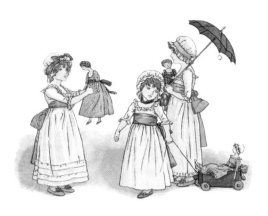

First Christmas

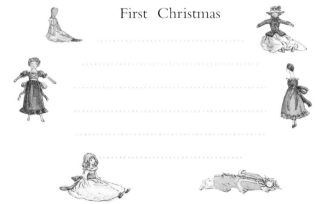

FIRST POSSESSIONS

First beaker

First bowl

First spoon

First mug or cup

First shoes

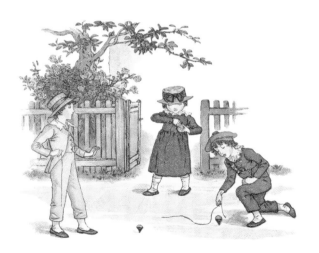

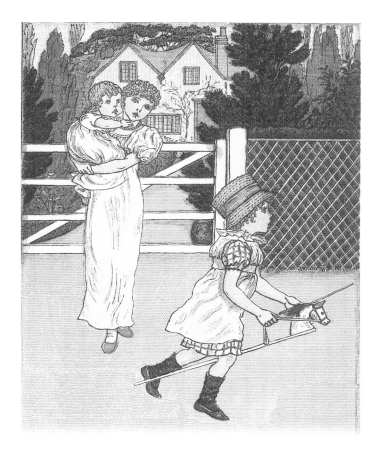

FIRST BIRTHDAY

Cake

Presents

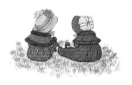

Relatives

Guests

Thoughts and feelings

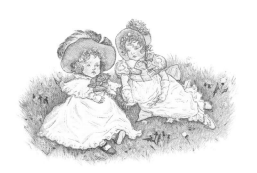

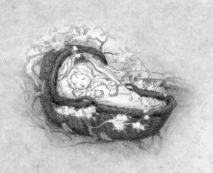